RAND

Evaluation of a Medicaid-Eligibility Expansion in Florida

Developing the Database

Ellen R. Harrison, Stephen H. Long,
M. Susan Marquis

Supported by the
Health Care Financing Administration,
    U.S. Department of Health and Human Services
March of Dimes Birth Defects Foundation

Preface

This report documents the construction of the analytic database used in a study of the 1989 Medicaid-eligibility expansion for pregnant women in Florida. It should be of interest to those who wish to link information from multiple data sources to study birth outcomes.

The research was supported by a cooperative agreement from the Health Care Financing Administration and a grant from the March of Dimes Birth Defects Foundation. Many people in Florida assisted in providing data and helping us understand the files—including Dan Thompson and Meade Grigg of the Department of Health and Rehabilitative Services and Fred Roberson and Jack Shi of the Medicaid program. The authors thank Robert Bell and Jeannette Rogowski for helpful comments on an earlier draft.

The analytic results of the study can be found in unpublished RAND research by Stephen H. Long and M. Susan Marquis on the effects of the Florida Medicaid-eligibility expansion for pregnant women.

Contents

Tables

Summary

To examine the effects of the 1989 Medicaid-eligibility expansion for pregnant women in Florida, we constructed a linked person-level database that contained information from eight different files. This report describes each of the sources and then details the linking procedure and the resulting analytic database.

We used two Vital Statistics files (VS) to define the universe of Florida deliveries. The birth certificate file and the fetal death file contained demographic information about the mother and baby as well as prenatal care and birth outcome data. The birth certificate file was linked to the death certificate file to identify babies who died within the first year of life.

We matched the VS records to the Hospital Discharge file to obtain insurance information. We developed a matching algorithm using hospital, patient's date of birth, date of first procedure, and patient's zip code. Approximately 88 percent of the VS records linked to a mother's discharge record according to our match criteria.

Using Social Security number, we matched the linked file to two additional files to obtain supplemental information for those using the public health system and those who were eligible for Medicaid. Seventy-six percent of women with prenatal care records on the Public Health System Encounter file matched to the linked file. Eighty percent of those identified as Medicaid on the linked file matched to a Social Security number on the Medicaid-Eligibility file.

Hospital characteristics were added for the 98 percent of cases we matched to the American Hospital Association database. Socioeconomic characteristics of the mother's neighborhood were included for the 95 percent of women with zip codes that matched to the 1990 census.

Our matching algorithm required exact matches when linkage variables were unique, such as Social Security number. It was more lenient for variables that are coded less reliably, such as zip code. This approach allowed us to maintain confidence in the reliability of the data without sacrificing the sample size. The final analysis files were rich with information from many sources and contained an average of 83 percent of the original population of births and fetal deaths.

1. Introduction

This report documents the construction of the analytic database used in a study of the 1989 Medicaid-eligibility expansion for pregnant women in Florida.[1] The creation of this database was a key challenge in the research. The resulting procedures may serve as a model for other evaluations of the Medicaid expansions.

The Medicaid-eligibility expansions for pregnant women and children were the most important policy changes in the program in the 1980s. Yet there are only a limited number of studies of the effects of these expansions, and it is not clear from these studies whether the expansions led to an improvement in prenatal care and birth outcomes.[2] Moreover, to understand the full effects of the interventions, it is also essential to understand how the Medicaid program changes affected other government programs that deliver prenatal care and how the expansions affected private payers. The effects on prenatal care access and birth outcomes are likely to be quite different if Medicaid-financed care substitutes for care previously financed and provided under other programs, such as Title V or private insurance, rather than providing new coverage for those who previously lacked insurance or access to other public programs. None of the previous studies, however, addresses these substitutions.

The objectives of our study were to investigate these interactions between the Medicaid program and other sources of financing and providing maternal health care and, with this perspective, to study whether pregnant women newly entitled to Medicaid coverage received more or earlier prenatal care, and whether their maternal and birth outcomes were improved. We studied the experience in Florida. Florida is a good site for this study for a number of reasons. It ranks fourth among the states in total population, and there are about 200,000 births there each year. Florida significantly expanded Medicaid eligibility for pregnant women and also aggressively implemented other strategies to ensure that women who were made eligible by the expansions gained coverage under the program. Florida relies heavily on county public health department clinics to

---

[1]Stephen H. Long and M. Susan Marquis, *The Effects of the Florida Medicaid Eligibility Expansion for Pregnant Women*, Final Report to Health Care Financing Administration and March of Dimes Birth Defects Foundation, December 1995.

[2]Alpha Center, *The Medicaid Expansions for Pregnant Women and Children*, Washington, D.C.: Alpha Center, 1995.

provide prenatal care to its low-income women, and hence it is a good place to study interactions between the Medicaid financing changes and the publicly financed direct-delivery system.

To conduct our analysis, we constructed a linked person-level database for the years 1988 through 1991 from vital statistics records, hospital discharge abstracts, public health system encounter data, Medicaid eligibility files, American Hospital Association annual survey data, and zip code–level data from the 1990 Census. This report first briefly describes the content of each database and then details our file linkage procedures and results.

2. The Data

Vital Statistics Data (VS)

Source: **Florida Department of Health and Rehabilitative Services**
Years: **1988–1991**

The VS contain information obtained from birth certificates, fetal death certificates, and death certificates from 1988 through 1991. They provide a detailed record of every birth and fetal death in the state of Florida for those years and define our study universe. Table 1 presents the total number of birth certificates and fetal death records in each of the study years. To determine the actual number of *women who delivered* in Florida, we subtracted the 1.2 percent of certificates that correspond to additional certificates for the same delivery (multiple births) and also excluded the births that took place outside of Florida. For example in 1991, the 195,756 certificates correspond to 193,393 mothers. After subtracting the out-of-state deliveries, we are left with 193,292 deliveries in the state of Florida.

The records include information about the pregnancy, such as the initiation and frequency of prenatal care, measures of birth outcomes such as birth weight and complications of delivery, and demographic characteristics of the mother and baby. Table 2 presents the key variables for analysis and for linking the VS with other databases. Because the mother's Social Security number is unique, universally used, and was included on over 95 percent of the VS records, it is the primary linkage variable for matching to the public health and Medicaid data. The mother's date of birth, name, and zip code as well as the hospital identification number were also used to link to other files.

The infant death records enable us to identify those infants who did not survive the first year of life. An infant death file for each year includes babies born during the year who died within the following 12 months. For 1988 and 1989, we were provided with a matched file in which the Florida Department of Health and Rehabilitative Services had linked the death certificate information with the birth certificates. For 1990 and 1991, we created the linked file, which combined information from the infant death file and the birth certificate file by matching death certificate numbers, when available, or by matching mother's and baby's name and baby's date of birth. We were able to match 97.5 percent of the 1990

4

Table 1

Live Births and Fetal Deaths from Vital Statistics Data, 1988–1991

Year	Live Births	Fetal Deaths	Total Certificates
1988	185,034	1,772	186,806
1989	193,893	1,833	195,726
1990	200,334	1,847	202,181
1991	194,043	1,713	195,756

Table 2

**Key Patient-Level Variables for Analysis and
Matching from Vital Statistics Files**

Mother's Characteristics
    Name
    Social Security number
    Date of birth
    Zip code of residence
    Race
    Educational attainment
    Marital status
Baby's Characteristics
    Name
    Birth weight
    Gestational age
    Sex
    Congenital anomalies
Pregnancy/Delivery Characteristics
    Mother smoked while pregnant
    Mother consumed alcohol while pregnant
    Number of previous births
    Singleton/multiple birth
    Month in which prenatal care began
    Number of prenatal care visits
    Labor complications
    Delivery complications

infant mortality records and 95.3 percent of the 1991 records. Table 3 presents the number of infant deaths and the infant mortality rate by year.

Hospital Discharge Data (HDD)

Source: Florida Agency for Health Care Administration
Years: 1988–1991

The HDD contain hospital discharge records from all nonmilitary acute care hospitals in Florida. We matched records of the mother's delivery hospitalization in this file with records from the VS file to obtain a number of key

Table 3

Vital Statistics–Linked Births and Infant Deaths, 1988–1991

	Infant Deaths	Percentage of Live Births
1988	1,892	1.02
1989	1,871	0.97
1990	1,883	0.94
1991[a]	1,441	0.74

[a]We did not have access to 1992 deaths, so the 1991 infant deaths represent just those infants who died in 1991.

variables that were not available from other sources. Most important to our analysis was the insurance status variable, which was defined as the principal payer for the hospitalization and had the following values:

- Medicaid
- Medicare
- Private
- Other.

The category "other" includes uninsured, charity, Champus, Veterans Administration, and other government third-party payers except Medicaid. We also collected primary diagnostic code, four secondary diagnostic codes, procedure codes, and the total charges for the delivery. The only person-level identifiers available to us were sex and date of birth.

We obtained all discharge records that had a maternity-related principal or secondary diagnosis.[1] Table 4 presents the number of discharge records on the resulting HDD file.

Public Health System Encounter Data (PH)

Source: **Florida Department of Health and Rehabilitative Services**
Years: **1987–1991**

The PH include information about each public health system client and his or her visits to public health department clinics from 1987 through 1991. We included

---

[1]ICD-9 codes 630–634, 638–676, V22–V24, V27, V28, V30–V39 were used to select the pregnancy and childbirth codes. We received guidance from an obstetrician to identify the codes generally associated with the actual delivery and also used the fifth-digit subclassification for codes 640–676 to separate out the delivery episode from the antepartum and postpartum episodes.

Table 4

HDD Maternity-Related Discharge Records, 1988–1991

	1988	1989	1990	1991
Pregnancy related	24,364	24,764	23,386	21,442
Delivery related	185,493	193,751	199,145	191,482

the 1987 data to capture all of the prenatal care visits for births occurring in the first part of 1988. We received over 13 million records for the five years of data, so our first task was to select all the prenatal care records—defined as visits that the health department identifies with the program component providing prenatal care (the Improved Pregnancy Outcome Program) and pregnancy tests provided by the Family Planning Program. We identified roughly 4 million prenatal care records. We linked all of the prenatal care visits for each woman into a single episode of prenatal care. For each episode, we constructed measures of the number of PH visits and the trimester in which prenatal care in the public health system was initiated.

Individuals are identified in the PH system using Social Security number, but 6 percent of the cases did not have valid values. Because we matched the PH to the VS file, we kept only those episodes with valid Social Security numbers. Table 5 presents the number of prenatal care episodes and total number of encounters per year, where year represents the ending date of the prenatal care episode. The end date was determined by either the presence of a postpartum visit or a lapse of more than 90 days between visits. In both cases, the end date was set to the previous visit.

Table 5

PH Prenatal Care Episodes and Total Visits, 1987–1991

Year	No. of Episodes	Total No. of Visits
1987	35,243	109,418
1988	43,115	185,495
1989	48,817	263,995
1990	62,646	331,932
1991[a]	83,299	497,076

[a]The numbers of 1991 episodes and visits are artificially high because they include some prenatal care episodes for births occurring in 1992.

Medicaid Eligibility Data (ME)

Source: **Florida Agency for Health Care Administration**
Years: **1988–1991**

The ME file we received from the Florida Agency for Health Care Administration was extracted to provide us with a complete account of periods of eligibility for women of childbearing age (12 through 55) who were enrolled in Medicaid at some time during 1988 through 1991. It was important to match this file to our other data sources to verify the insurance status of the mother from the HDD file, to determine the reason for eligibility, and to examine the timing of the eligibility relative to the pregnancy. After selecting the 99 percent of records with valid Social Security numbers, to match to the other databases, and those with eligibility periods that included any portion of our study years, we had roughly 1.3 million records for the study period. Table 6 presents the total number of eligibility records for each of the years.

The ME files contain name, Social Security number, Medicaid identification number, the periods of Medicaid eligibility, and the basis of Medicaid entitlement for each eligibility period. We categorized the basis of entitlement into the following groups:

- Aid to Families with Dependent Children (AFDC)
- Medically needy
- Expansion group below 100 percent of poverty
- Expansion group between 100 and 150 percent of poverty
- Other.

Table 6

**Medicaid Eligibility Records,
1988–1991**

Year	No. of Eligibility Records
1988	240,905
1989	297,347
1990	364,960
1991	387,817

American Hospital Association Annual Survey of Hospitals (AHA)

Source: **American Hospital Association**
Year: **1991**

The 1991 American Hospital Association Annual Survey of Hospitals contains hospital characteristics for all participating hospitals in the United States, including 306 Florida hospitals. We supplemented the file with information from the 1988 AHA guide for nine hospitals in our files that either closed or merged with other hospitals prior to 1991.[2]

Our primary use of these data was to measure the ownership of each hospital in which each delivery occurred. The variable has the following categories:

- Government, nonfederal
- Nongovernment, nonprofit
- Nongovernment, proprietary
- Federal.

We also used these data to measure delivery-specific characteristics of each hospital such as number of births, number of newborn days, and presence of a neonatal intensive care unit, as well as general information concerning the type of hospital, number of beds, number of Medicaid admissions, intern- and resident-to-bed ratio, and total facility and hospital-unit expenses.

Census of Population and Housing Summary Data (CEN)

Source: **Bureau of the Census**
Year: **1990**

The Census Bureau produces a summary tape (*Summary Tape File 3B*) for the Census of Population and Housing that provides summary information aggregated to the zip code level for all persons and housing units in the United States. We created an extract of the 826 Florida zip codes that existed in 1990. Because we did not have a measure of income for the women in the study, we used incomes in the residence area as a proxy measure. The CEN file was used to calculate the percentage of zip code residents falling into different income

---

[2] Births in these 315 hospitals accounted for over 98 percent of all births in nonmilitary, nonmaternity Florida hospitals over the study period.

categories expressed as a percentage of the federal poverty level.[3] By merging these data to the VS file, we constructed a proxy measure of income for each woman giving birth in a year based on the percentage of the population in the zip code of residence with a family income below 150 percent of poverty.

---

[3]The income information was collected for approximately one in six households covered by the 1990 census.

3. Matching Procedures

Linking Hospital Discharge Data to the Vital Statistics

Matching Algorithm

The primary challenge in the linkage process was to match the vital statistics record of a birth with the mother's hospital discharge record in the absence of a unique identifier on the hospital discharge data. Our algorithm matched by hospital first, and then within hospital, by mother's date of birth, baby's date of birth, and mother's zip code of residence.

Both files had a hospital identifier, but because the two sources used different coding schemes, we used county and hospital name in our matching algorithm. After modifying the two lists to have standard abbreviations and punctuation, we matched by county and the first eight letters of the hospital name. This task was complicated by hospitals that changed names, merged with other hospitals, or closed during the study years. To aid in our matching of hospitals with similar names, we made separate calculations from the two files of the number of births occurring at each hospital and then compared the totals from the potential matches.

For each of the four study years, roughly 94 percent of the births on the VS file occurred at hospitals that were candidates to match to the HDD file. Over 40 percent of the noncandidate births took place at military hospitals, while another 20 percent were performed at maternity centers. Neither type of facility is included on the HDD database. Table 7 presents the distribution of location of births by year. The top row represents the percentage of cases that were eligible for the next step of the matching algorithm.

Once we made a hospital-level match, we used a patient-level matching algorithm. We first identified the variables that were common to both files— birth date of patient and zip code of residence. The mother's HDD discharge record also included the date of first surgical procedure, which is almost always the delivery date and thus could be used as a proxy for the baby's birth date. This additional linking variable increased our ability to find unique matches and increased our confidence in the validity of the match. The third data element, zip

Table 7

Distribution of Location of VS Live Births and Fetal Deaths, by Year
(in percentage)

Location	1988	1989	1990	1991
HDD hospital	94.4	94.6	94.1	94.7
Military hospital	2.5	2.2	2.4	2.4
Maternity center	0.9	1.1	1.2	1.3
Nonhospital	0.7	0.7	0.6	0.6
Out of Florida	0.6	0.5	0.5	0.1
Enroute to hospital	0.2	0.2	0.2	0.1
Unknown	0.7	0.8	0.9	0.9

code of residence, was available on 99 percent of both the VS and HDD files. We used a hierarchical approach in which we first required a match on all three linking variables, then subsequently loosened the restrictions requiring either an exact match on mother's birth date and baby's birth date with missing or nonmatching zip codes, or else a match on mother's birth date and zip code with the baby's birth falling sometime within the time of hospitalization, although not on the procedure date.

Using this algorithm, we were able to match between 91 percent and 94 percent of the VS events that occurred at an HDD hospital. If we use the entire universe of VS births and fetal deaths as the denominator, the match rate ranges from 86 percent for 1988 to 89 percent for 1991. Among VS records that had matched to the HDD at the hospital level, the percentage satisfying each of the match criteria, as well as those that remain unmatched, are shown in Table 8.

If we had limited our definition of a successful match to only those instances in which there was agreement on all three linkage variables, our match rate would

Table 8

VS Match Rate to HDD File, 1988–1991
(in percentage)

	1988	1989	1990	1991
Match on mother's dob, baby's dob, zip code	73.5	74.1	76.9	77.3
Match on mother's dob, baby's dob (not zip code)	12.7	11.1	10.6	11.0
Match on mother's dob & zip code, birth w/in hospitalization	5.1	7.6	6.7	6.2
Unmatched VS record (w/match at hospital level)	8.8	7.2	5.7	5.5

NOTE: dob is date of birth.

have decreased to an average of 75 percent of the eligible VS records. We felt that it was important to allow for some disagreement in variables that either tend to have missing values or are coded less reliably, such as zip code. Similarly, because procedure date is not a perfect proxy for the baby's birth date, it was reasonable to allow some leeway.

Alternatively, we could have increased our match rate by loosening our restrictions or by adding a step in which records were compared manually. The former approach would have decreased the reliability of the data to a point where we would begin to lose confidence in the data. The latter approach of taking the time to manually compare lists of records to pick up a few additional matches was a trade-off that we rejected given the immense size of the databases and the high match rate we were able to achieve using a completely automated approach.

Duplicate Matches

Our confidence in the matching algorithm was bolstered because, on average, 97 percent of the VS records corresponding to deliveries in HDD hospitals had a one-to-one exact match to a record on the HDD file. The non-unique matches resulted from two factors: (1) multiple births and (2) records for more than one mother in one source matching to one or more records in the other source.

Approximately 2.3 percent of babies born each year were part of multiple births. These cases had a birth certificate for each baby but only one mother's discharge record. Because our unit of analysis was the delivery rather than the birth, we selected one of the birth certificates at random to be used in the analyses.

The remainder of the non-unique matches occurred because two or more records from at least one of the VS and HDD files had identical values for hospital, mother's birthday/age, baby's birthday and zip code of residence. This problem was more prevalent in 1988 when the VS file recorded mother's age in years rather than by the more precise birth date.

In the 1989–1991 files, less than 0.2 percent of the records in both VS and HDD had nondiscriminating match values in each year. However, in 1988 close to 3 percent of the VS records were non-unique; 1 percent matched a single record in the HDD file, and close to 2 percent matched to multiple HDD records. As one might expect, the hospitals with the highest volume of deliveries were most susceptible to this problem. The five hospitals with at least 5,000 deliveries in 1988 accounted for 21 percent of all deliveries and 30 percent of the nonexact matches.

We had no additional information with which to determine the correct match, so we examined the length of stay, total charge, and payer variables from the candidate HDD records. In most instances, the length of stay and charge values were comparable, and in more than half the cases, the payer value was the same. Because (1) most of the variables used for the analysis come from the VS file, (2) the Medicaid status is verified when matched to the ME file, and (3) the cases represented a small proportion of the data, we opted for a simple resolution. When one or more VS record matched to multiple HDD records, we randomly assigned the match among the candidate discharge records. For the few cases when multiple VS records matched to one HDD record, we matched both records to the same discharge. The final analysis sample included one match per VS record so that it represented the number of deliveries in Florida as recorded by the VS.

Unmatched HDD Records

Although we used the VS file to define our universe, we also examined the nonmatching HDD records. An average of 13 percent of HDD records identified as delivery discharges did not match to the VS file. We compared the diagnostic codes for the nonmatches with the matching records to determine how they differed. Over one-third of the nonmatches had a primary diagnosis of abortion or ectopic pregnancy and thus should not have been expected to match to the VS file. Less than 0.1 percent of the matches had a similar diagnostic code.

The remaining number of nonmatches is only slightly higher than the number of VS nonmatches that took place in HDD hospitals. This difference could be attributed to nonresidents who delivered in Florida hospitals and thus would be on the HDD but not on the VS file. Table 9 presents the match rates by year.

Linking in Medicaid Eligibility Data

The VS and ME both contain Social Security number and mother's date of birth. We linked the files by mother's Social Security number and then verified the match by comparing the date-of-birth values. For each study year, approximately 95 percent of the VS records had valid Social Security numbers and were candidates for matching.

Because the ME had one record for each period of Medicaid eligibility, after matching by Social Security number, we needed to identify which eligibility period contained the date of baby's birth to correctly measure whether the

Table 9

Match Rate for HDD Records, 1988–1991

	1988	1989	1990	1991
Match to VS	157,620	167,642	173,671	169,069
	(85 percent)	(87 percent)	(87 percent)	(88 percent)
Unmatched	27,873	25,929	25,474	22,413
	(15 percent)	(13 percent)	(13 percent)	(12 percent)

mother was covered at the time of delivery and the basis of entitlement at that time.

Of the HDD records with valid Social Security numbers and with Medicaid as the primary payer, approximately 80 percent matched to an eligibility record on the ME file. Table 10 presents the match rate by year.

Although the key reason for linking to the ME file was to identify the basis of Medicaid entitlement, the match to the eligibility file also enabled us to identify the potential false positives—women identified as being covered by Medicaid on the HDD but not eligible at the time of delivery on the ME file.[1] Because the Medicaid file is used as an official source for identifying Medicaid eligibles and screening claims for payment, we used the ME data to resolve discrepancies between it and the HDD.

For 1991, we were also able to examine the false negatives—Medicaid-eligible mothers not identified on the HDD as having a Medicaid payer—by linking to the Medicaid inpatient hospital claims data (MC). Claims data with delivery diagnosis codes were used for this investigation to determine the number of Medicaid mothers who had deliveries—that is, the denominator for the estimate of false negatives. These records were matched back to the ME using the

Table 10

Percentage of Medicaid HDD Matching to ME File

Year	Percentage
1988	67
1989	73
1990	79
1991	92

---

[1]A small number of the "false positives" could be the Medicaid medically needy who were not Medicaid eligible at admission but, because of complications, accrued enough charges during the hospitalization to become eligible prior to discharge. We do not have enough information to identify these spend-down cases but believe they would account for a small percentage of those we identified as false positives.

Medicaid identification number, and were then linked to the VS file using the method above. Eighty-five percent of the delivery claims on the MC file successfully matched to the VS file.

Linking in Public Health System Encounter Data

Because the dates in the PH are dates for prenatal care visits, there was no exact date we could use to match to the baby's date of birth on the VS file. However, we could not ignore date altogether because a number of women gave birth multiple times within the study period. In addition, roughly 120 women per year appear on the VS file as having delivered twice within the same year.

To ensure that the episode was matched to the correct delivery, we developed a two-stage algorithm. We first matched on mother's Social Security number and the year of baby's birth where we used the end of the prenatal care episode to define the PH value for year (except for episodes ending in 1987 that were coded as 1988 to match to the earliest births in our study). If the birth date occurred prior to the first prenatal care visit or later than six months after the last visit, the birth year value on the PH record was recoded to one year later, and the second stage of the match was performed using mother's Social Security number and the alternate birth year.

To accurately count the total number of PH visits associated with deliveries, we needed to estimate what percentage of the records corresponded to a birth during the study years. By examining the records that matched to the VS file, we used the relationship between the last date of prenatal care and the year of delivery to simulate the delivery year for the records we were unable to match. For example, 14 percent of the prenatal care episodes ending in October 1990 matched to a delivery in 1991, so we estimated that 14 percent of the unmatched records ending in October 1990 corresponded to births that occurred in 1991. Because we did not have access to 1992 records, we also estimated that 14 percent of the October 1991 episodes corresponded to births outside of the study period. Assigning unmatched records in this way, between 73 and 81 percent of the PH prenatal care visits that corresponded to a delivery in 1988 to 1991 were matched to the VS file. Table 11 presents the match rate for the PH records by the year of delivery.

Table 11

**Percentage of PH Prenatal Care Visits
Matched to VS File, by Year**

Year	Percentage
1988	77
1989	81
1990	74
1991	73

Linking in American Hospital Association Annual Survey of Hospitals Data

The AHA file's hospital identification number was different from both the VS and HDD identifiers. We used the same algorithm that was used for the hospital-level match between the VS and HDD files, although we could now compare the AHA name with both the VS *and* HDD version of the hospital name. After most matches were made using an automated routine comparing the first letters of the hospital names, the few remaining cases were examined manually to identify the correct match. Of the 306 hospitals on the AHA file, all but 12 matched to either a VS or HDD hospital. An examination of the "number of births" variable from the AHA file revealed that none of the unmatched hospitals had any deliveries.[2]

Linking in the Census of Population and Housing Summary Data

Of all the women on the VS file who gave birth between 1988 and 1991, 95 percent of them lived in the 825 zip codes that matched to the CEN file. Of the VS cases that did not match, 86 percent had zip codes that were in the range of Florida values but were either mispunches or zip codes that did not exist at the time the CEN file was created. The nonmatches were retained on the file and set to missing. The 825 matched zip codes accounted for all but one of the zip codes on the CEN file.

The Final Linked File

The final linked file contains one VS record per delivery and includes only those that matched to a HDD record. Table 12 presents the original number of records

---

[2]Approximately 2 percent of births occurred in military hospitals or maternity centers that were not included in the AHA file.

Table 12

Comparison of Original VS File to Matched Files, by Year

	1988	1989	1990	1991
Number of deliveries on VS file[a]	184,798	193,336	199,663	193,393
Match to HDD (final linked file)	159,077 (86 percent)	169,548 (88 percent)	177,153 (89 percent)	173,033 (89 percent)
Match HDD and AHA	157,217 (85 percent)	167,587 (87 percent)	174,491 (87 percent)	170,758 (88 percent)
Match HDD, AHA, and CEN	145,203 (79 percent)	158,622 (82 percent)	168,498 (84 percent)	165,333 (85 percent)

[a]Total number of deliveries includes deliveries to residents that took place outside of Florida.

and then the number and percentage of records with successful matches to the HDD, AHA, and CEN files, cumulatively. Thus the final linked file is composed of records that represent between 86 and 89 percent of the deliveries to Florida mothers between 1988 and 1991.[3] In addition, we were able to match between 79 and 85 percent of the VS cases to the HDD, AHA, and CEN files—the three link files that were applicable to all of the records. The final linked file also includes the additional information obtained for the subset of Medicaid eligible and low-income women by matching to the ME and PH files.

_____

[3]Because 4 to 5 percent of the records in the final linked file have missing values for some of the key outcome measures or demographic characteristics, an analysis file containing only those records with complete data would be slightly smaller.

4. Conclusion

By using different variables to link multiple files, we were able to create a database rich with information from multiple sources. The payer information from the HDD, the detailed prenatal care data from the PH, and the eligibility criteria from the Medicaid file (ME) added person-specific details that could not be obtained from the VS. In addition, links to the AHA and Census file provided us with useful control variables at the hospital and zip code level. Our matching algorithm included verification measures at each step so that we could be confident in the accuracy of the matches without forfeiting the sample size. Because there is often a wealth of information collected, but not from one source, such techniques are necessary to construct the most complete analytic database possible.